Calm and Clear

KNEAD YOUR WAY TO ZEN

by Rebekah Borucki

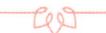

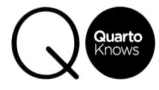

Brimming with creative inspiration, how-to projects, and useful information to enrich your everyday life, Quarto Knows is a favorite destination for those pursuing their interests and passions. Visit our site and dig deeper with our books into your area of interest: Quarto Creates, Quarto Cooks, Quarto Homes, Quarto Lives, Quarto Drives, Quarto Explores, Quarto Gifts, or Quarto Kids.

© 2019 Quarto Publishing Group USA Inc.

Published in 2019 by becker&mayer! books, an imprint of The Quarto Group, 11120 NE 33rd Place, Suite 201, Bellevue, WA 98004 USA.
www.QuartoKnows.com

This book is part of the *Calm and Clear* kit and is not to be sold separately.

becker&mayer! books titles are also available at discount for retail, wholesale, promotional, and bulk purchase. For details, contact the Special Sales Manager by email at specialsales@quarto.com or by mail at The Quarto Group, Attn: Special Sales Manager, 100 Cummings Center Suite 265D, Beverly, MA 01915 USA.

19 20 21 22 23   5 4 3 2 1

ISBN: 978-0-7603-6760-5

Library of Congress Cataloging-in-Publication Data available upon request.

Author: Rebekah Borucki
Design: Lauren Clulow
Photography: Chris Burrows
Editorial: Bonnie Honeycutt
Production: Michael Nash & Blake Mitchum

Printed, manufactured, and assembled in Shenzhen, China, 08/19.

Distributed by:
Quarto UK, The Old Brewery
6 Blundell Street, London N7 9BH, UK
Allen & Unwin
30 Centre Rd, Scoresby VIC 3179, AUS

Image credits: All stock photographs and design elements © Shutterstock

#327396

This product contains wheat and natural lavender and rosemary essential oils.
Stop using product if you experience redness or irritation.
Seek medical attention if irritation persists.
Shelf life 09/2022.

TABLE OF CONTENTS

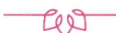

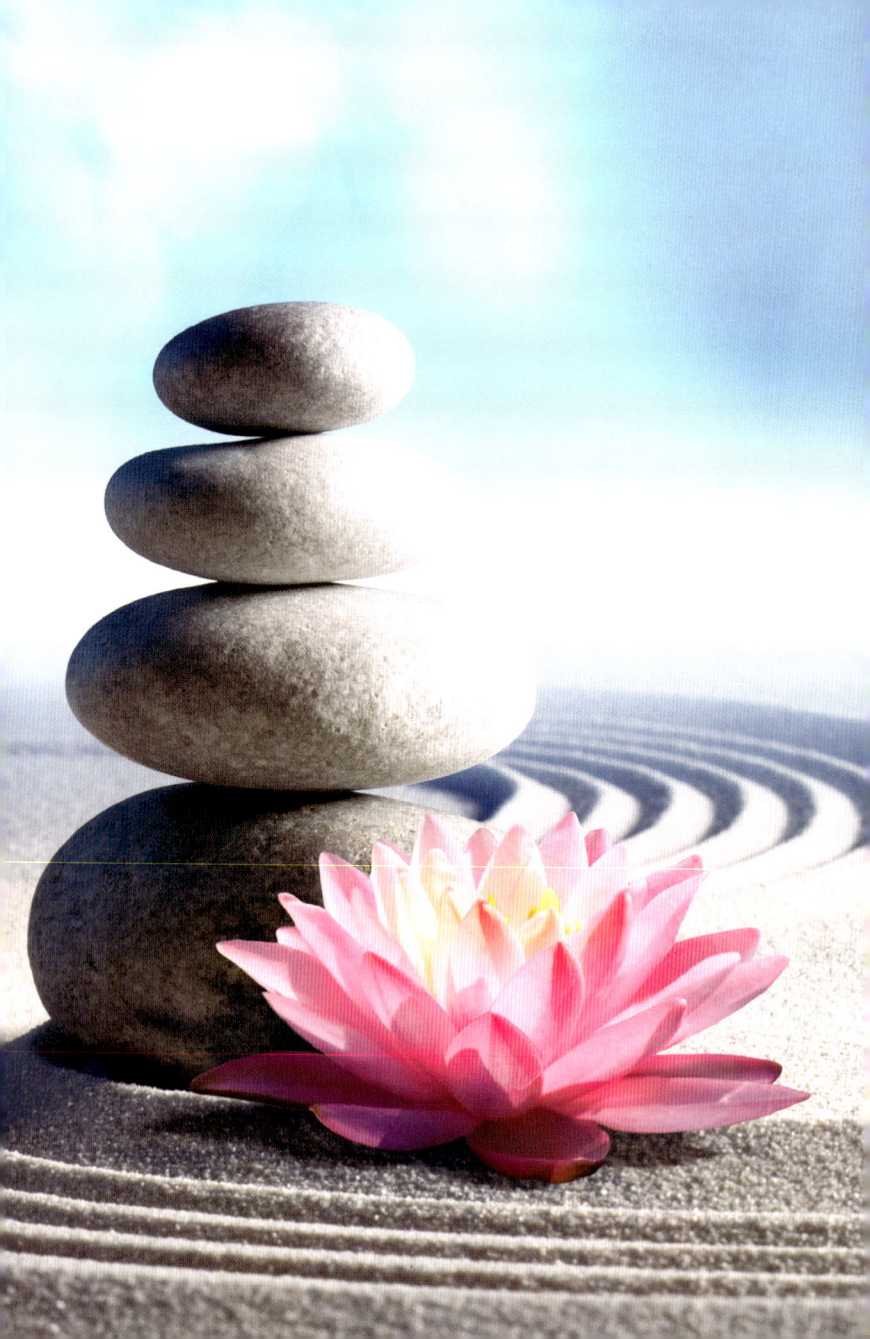

Introduction

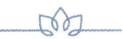

KNEAD YOUR
WAY TO ZEN

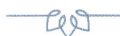

As our lives become busier and more stressful, the need for easy, accessible self-care tools begins to skyrocket. Meditation is a tried-and-true ancient method that brings balance to both the mind and body—a simple practice that's perfectly suited for the modern world. So it makes sense that you picked up this book to learn more about it.

An effective meditation practice can require as little as a quiet spot and the willingness of the practitioner to be alone with their thoughts for a few moments. If you can breathe, you can meditate. There are no special skills required.

However, there are elements you can add to enhance your practice. You're going to learn about several of those elements on the following pages. A set of two *Calm and Clear* scented doughs came with this book. You'll use them in combination with hand mudras—symbolic hand gestures—to enhance the physical part of your practice and to incorporate the power of aromatherapy into your time on the meditation pillow. A guide for creating positive affirmations, instructions for comfortable sitting positions, and a tutorial for beneficial breathing methods are also offered in easy-to-follow steps.

Many people desire balance, calm, clarity, and peace of mind, which can feel like an unattainable goal. Rest assured that all of these are attainable with just a little effort, made regularly and with a focused mind. Pay close attention to what's laid out for you in the lessons in this book, and practice what you learn. All the good feelings you've wished for are within reach.

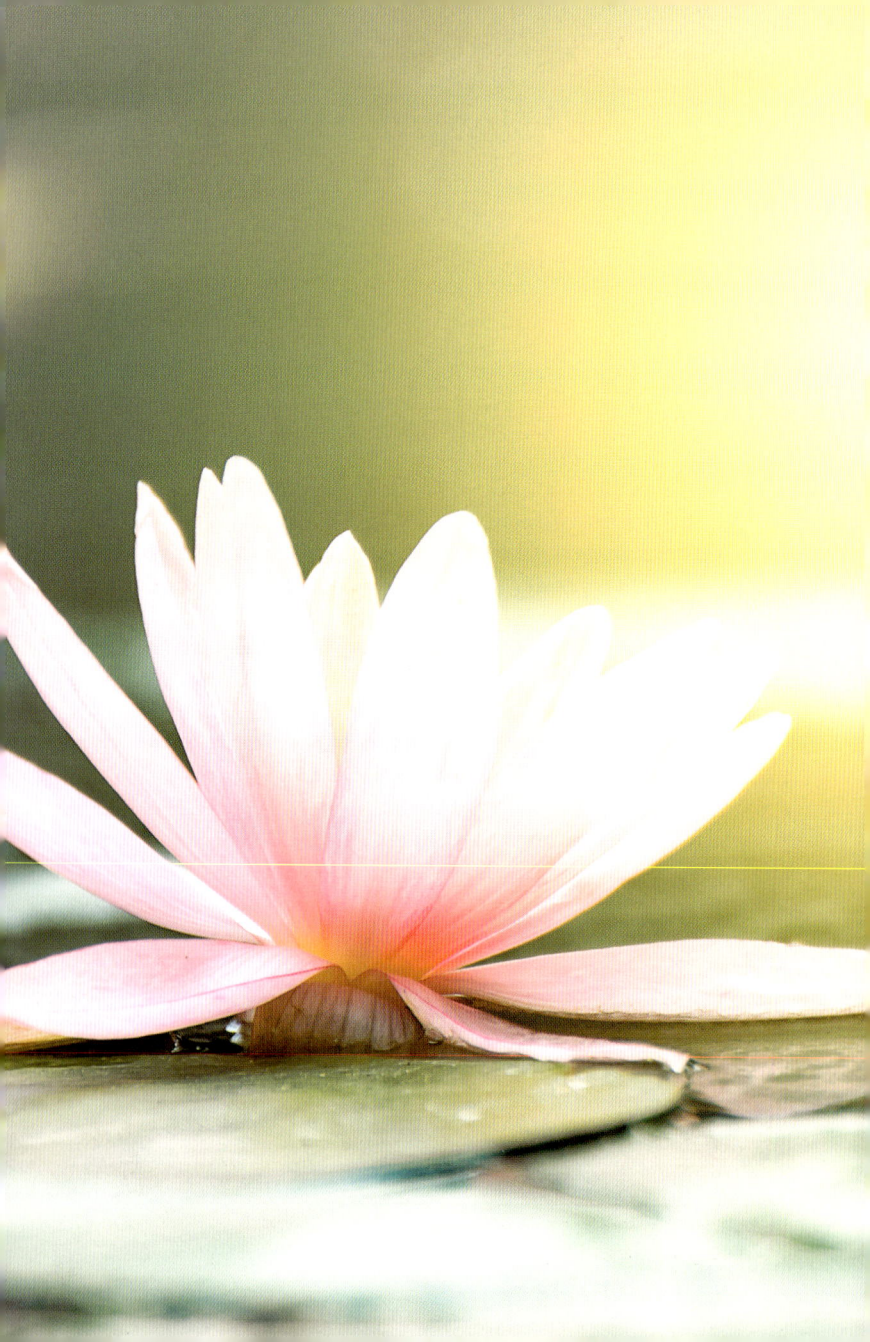

Chapter One

USING MANTRA
& MOVEMENT

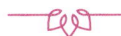

common concern for meditation is that a successful practice
requires clearing the mind of all thoughts. Making this the
goal will likely lead to frustration and, eventually, to giving up
altogether. It might take years or a lifetime of practice to think about
nothing. For now, it would be more helpful for you to approach meditation
as a practice in *focus* rather than a time to zone out into oblivion.

Still, focus may be difficult. We're all so busy nowadays, and the chaos
of life has tens of thousands of thoughts running through our heads on a
daily basis. Depending on the study, it's estimated that the human brain
processes between 12,000 and 70,000 thoughts per day. Picture them
as a train, traveling on a track in circles in and out of your conscious and
subconscious minds, never stopping or changing course.

Consider the impact of a message that's repeated over and over again—for example, a television commercial for a hot new product. Seeing the commercial only one time may have little or no effect on you, especially if the product doesn't particularly interest you. Now, imagine seeing that commercial dozens of times in a single day. After just a few views, you might start humming along with the jingle. After a few more, the song sticks in your head. If it's a commercial for a food product, images of the tasty treat might come to mind at your next mealtime. Before you know it, you're singing the jingle out loud, craving the product, and hunting for it in the grocery store.

Take a moment to think about all the product taglines, slogans, and jingles you've memorized over your lifetime. They're embedded in the deep recesses of your brain's memory centers. That's the power of a repeated message. What starts as a simple idea or message becomes a permanent fixture, a repeated narrative that we carry with us always.

That's the power of a repeated message.

What can be troubling about repeated thoughts is that many can be negative. Worry about a future event is a perfect example of negative repetitive thought. Human beings are great at creating negative stories about imaginary events. What was the last thing you were worried about? How many times have you replayed an undesirable scenario—something you didn't want to happen, but kept imagining it might—in your head? How did that make you feel? Certainly not calm, clear, or relaxed. It most likely made you feel anxious, confused, and overwhelmed.

So how do you keep repetitive thoughts from creeping into your head during meditation? How can you use the power of thoughts to your advantage? How do we become the conductor of our thought trains, so that they set course in a positive direction instead of turning into runaway disasters? The answer lies in the power of mantra.

What Is a Mantra?

....

Mantra is an ancient Sanskrit word for a sacred sound, word, or phrase that is repeated during meditation to aid in concentration.[1] Broken down into two parts, *man* is translated as *mind* and *tra* means *instrument* or *vehicle*. You can look at mantras as vehicles of the mind designed to get you to a meditative state faster and make the journey a pleasant one. A mantra can act as a "train of thought" carrying positive messages and feelings from your conscious mind into your subconscious mind, embedding them permanently into your psyche and changing the way you experience your environment.

When you repeat a single sound, word, or phrase in a rhythmic pattern, it draws your attention away from whatever else is happening and toward what's being repeated. Just as closing your eyes removes visual distractions, and covering your ear quiets audible disturbances, repeating mantras clears mental clutter. Using mantras puts you in the conductor's seat—it puts you in control.

Making Mantras Part of Your Practice

....

A positive affirmation can serve as a meditation mantra. Repeating an uplifting or motivational phrase can shift your mindset and even your physical state instantaneously. Positive words repeated as a mantra during meditation shift your focus to something that supports a state of peace and calm. Affirmative mantras are your ticket to a positive thought train that's traveling to a calmer, happier version of you.

Finding the right mantra for your meditation practice is simple. You can create your own or find one that's already written. A simple Internet search for motivational affirmations will deliver many good options. You can also search websites that serve as quote libraries. Typing words like "happiness" or "peace" into the search field will lead you to inspirational musings by great thinkers, celebrities, political and historical figures, and artists.

To create your own mantra, follow these four steps.

....

1. Identify your discomfort.

Think of a situation or emotion that you're struggling with. For example, you might have a conflict with a friend or worry about a financial issue.

2. Express your problem in a short sentence.

If you're worried about the fate of a relationship, you might say, "I'm scared of losing my best friend over a petty disagreement."

3. Give your best advice.

Imagine you're consoling a loved one who has come to you with the same concern. What's the first kind thing you would say to them? Maybe it would be, "You're a good person who deserves good people in your life. You should be honest with your feelings and trust that things will work out for the best."

4. Flip the script.

Creating a motivational, inspirational, or comforting mantra for yourself is as easy as giving yourself your best good advice. Take the words you would offer your loved one and make them yours. Always write your mantra in the present tense. It is an affirmation of the goodness that's available to you right now. "I'm a good person who deserves good people in my life. I can be honest with my feelings. I can trust that things will work out for the best." That's three separate positive mantras.

Whether you borrow a mantra from someone else or decide to make your own, make sure it's short and easy to remember. You'll repeat your mantra again and again throughout your meditation or whenever your attention drifts. It will allow you to return quickly to a focused meditative state.

How to Use the Dough

....

Many religions and spiritual traditions use beads to help with concentration and for counting prayers or mantras. For instance, Catholics use a strand of beads when they recite the rosary (a specific system of prayer), moving individual beads through their fingers as they finish one round of recitation and move on to the next. Similar practices are found in Hinduism, Buddhism, and other traditions. If you practice yoga, perhaps you are familiar with mala beads used for reciting mantras, made of 108 beads plus one "guru" bead.

Prayers and mantras differ between cultures, but the purpose of meditation beads is the same. They occupy the physical body by focusing the hands on a repetitive movement, helping the one who is praying or meditating stay focused on their task.

Engage your senses to create an experience that calms your body...

This book came with scented dough that you'll learn to use in your meditation practice. If you are wondering how dough is going to help you go deeper within and bring you closer to Zen, you might be surprised to learn that you've done something like this before. Chances are that you use meditative tools in many areas of your life to self-soothe and get into "the zone." Sitting still isn't the only way to practice meditation.

Maybe you're someone who enjoys cooking. Imagine yourself in the kitchen, standing over a big pot of wonderful-smelling stew, stirring in one direction and then another, observing how the contents of the pot swirl together. You get lost in the moment, tuning out all outside distractions, and find yourself focusing only on the task at hand. Similarly, rolling balls of cookie dough between your palms and placing them on a baking sheet can be a soothing practice at the end of a stressful day.

A walk outdoors is another way to focus your attention on the present moment. Engage your senses to create an experience that calms your body while also clearing your mind of negative, stressful, or distracting thoughts. Observe the colors, shapes, and tiny details of your surroundings with your eyes. Listen to the sound of leaves crunching beneath your feet, or your shoes hitting the pavement. Sink into the rhythm of your footsteps.

Examples of Ways to Knead the Dough

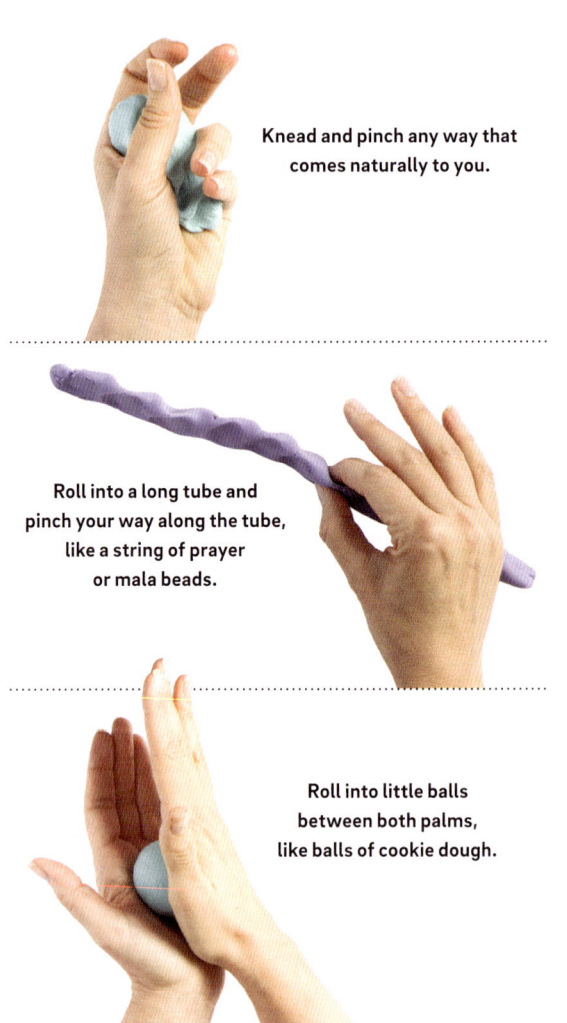

Knead and pinch any way that comes naturally to you.

Roll into a long tube and pinch your way along the tube, like a string of prayer or mala beads.

Roll into little balls between both palms, like balls of cookie dough.

An added benefit to using the scented dough is that the warmth of your hands release the aromatherapy. Use your scented dough to practice a moving meditation, much like you would use meditation beads. But don't worry—you'll only be making small movements with your hands, and you can do the whole meditation while sitting in whichever position is most comfortable for you. The easiest way to use the tools you've learned about so far is to repeat a few simple mantras while working the dough in your hands.

Let's keep it simple with a few short mantras for calming, clearing, and supporting a positive mindset. You'll learn more advanced breathing techniques in the next chapter, but for now, you're just going to use your natural breathing pattern to guide you.

Each of your mantras includes the words "I am." This two-word phrase is one of the most powerful mantras in the universe. Whatever follows it defines who you are or what you'd like to manifest at that moment. Always be mindful how you use "I am" in your everyday conversations—including self-talk. For instance, instead of saying "I am sick," try, "I am getting healthier and healthier with every breath I take." That certainly isn't a cure for everything that ails you, but it can help to keep you in a positive state of mind while dealing with the stress of not feeling well.

Use your scented dough to practice a moving meditation.

It's important to focus only on your mantra during your practice, so removing visual distractions is recommended. Close your eyes while repeating your mantras, or if that's uncomfortable for you, keep them open and focus on an image or object in front of you. Some suggestions for objects include a lit candle, flowers, or one of the inspirational photographs provided throughout this book.

Think of your mantras and scented dough as take-anywhere tools that can help you enter a state of peace and calm no matter the location, situation, or time of day. There's no need to set aside a lot of time for this practice. All you need is a few moments to close your eyes, connect with your breath, and recite a few supportive words. Tuck your dough in your bedside table drawer, your desk, or your bag. A sense of feeling calm and clear will always be just a few moments away.

🌸 **Mantra 1:** "I am safe. I am calm. I am at peace."

Use the lavender-scented dough for this mantra. Lavender is recommended for stress reduction and relaxation.[2] Sitting comfortably in a position that works for you, close your eyes and hold the dough in one or both of your hands. Keep your hands open with the dough resting in your upturned palms. As you inhale through your nose, gently close your hands and knead the dough, releasing the scent. On your exhale, open your hands and repeat your mantra either silently to yourself or out loud with a whisper. Inhale and knead. Exhale, and repeat your mantra while opening your hands. Repeat this cycle for as long as you'd like or for a total of ten rounds of inhales and exhales.

🌸 **Mantra 2:** "In this moment, I am choosing joy."

While lavender is used as a calming scent, rosemary is indicated for focus, clarity, and igniting the senses.[3] Depending on how you'd like to feel, you may use either dough with this mantra. Follow the same steps as before: Holding the dough in your upturned palms, inhale through your nose while kneading the dough. Then recite your mantra on your exhale while slowly opening your hands.

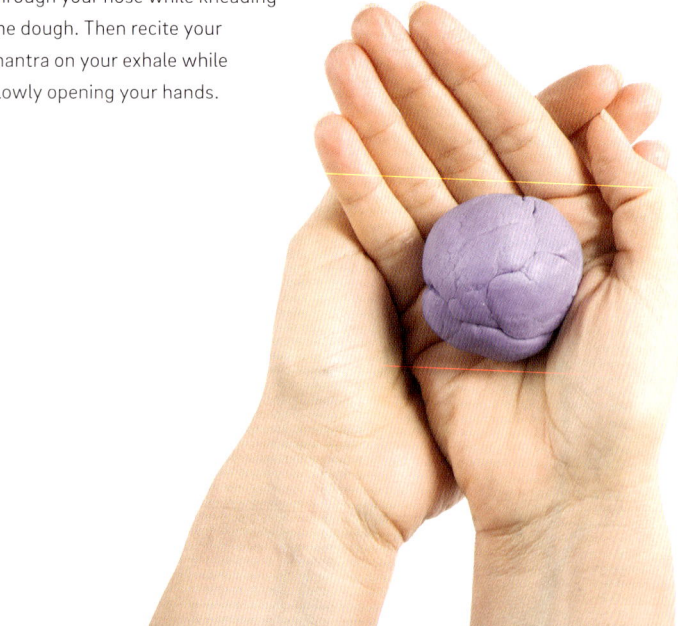

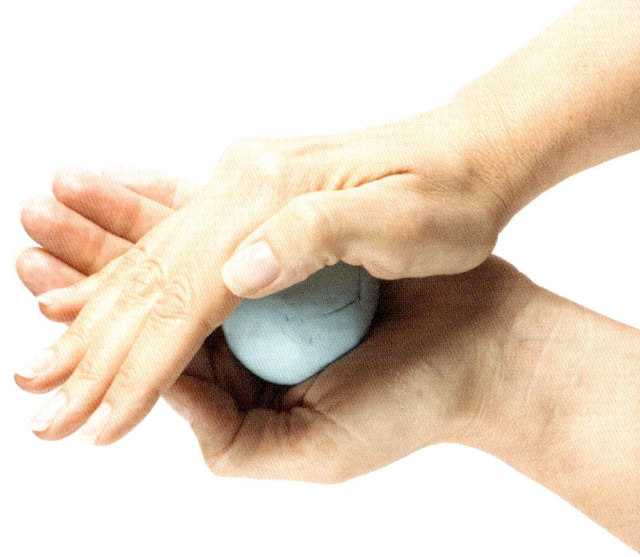

🏵 **Mantra 3:** "I am happy, healthy, and alive!"

Your rosemary-scented dough is ideal for this invigorating mantra. Add a twist to your practice by smiling as you repeat your mantra to help seal in all the good feelings it's delivering to every part of your body. Each breath cycle will help you to feel more awake, alert, and ready for whatever your day has in store for you. Be mindful not to practice with rosemary right before bed. That's a time for relaxation, not waking up your brain.

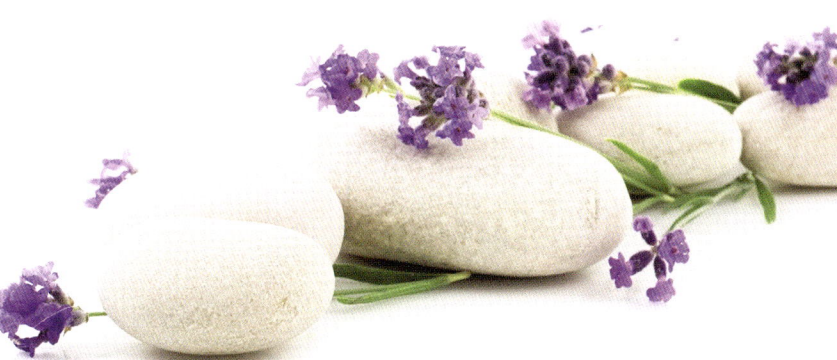

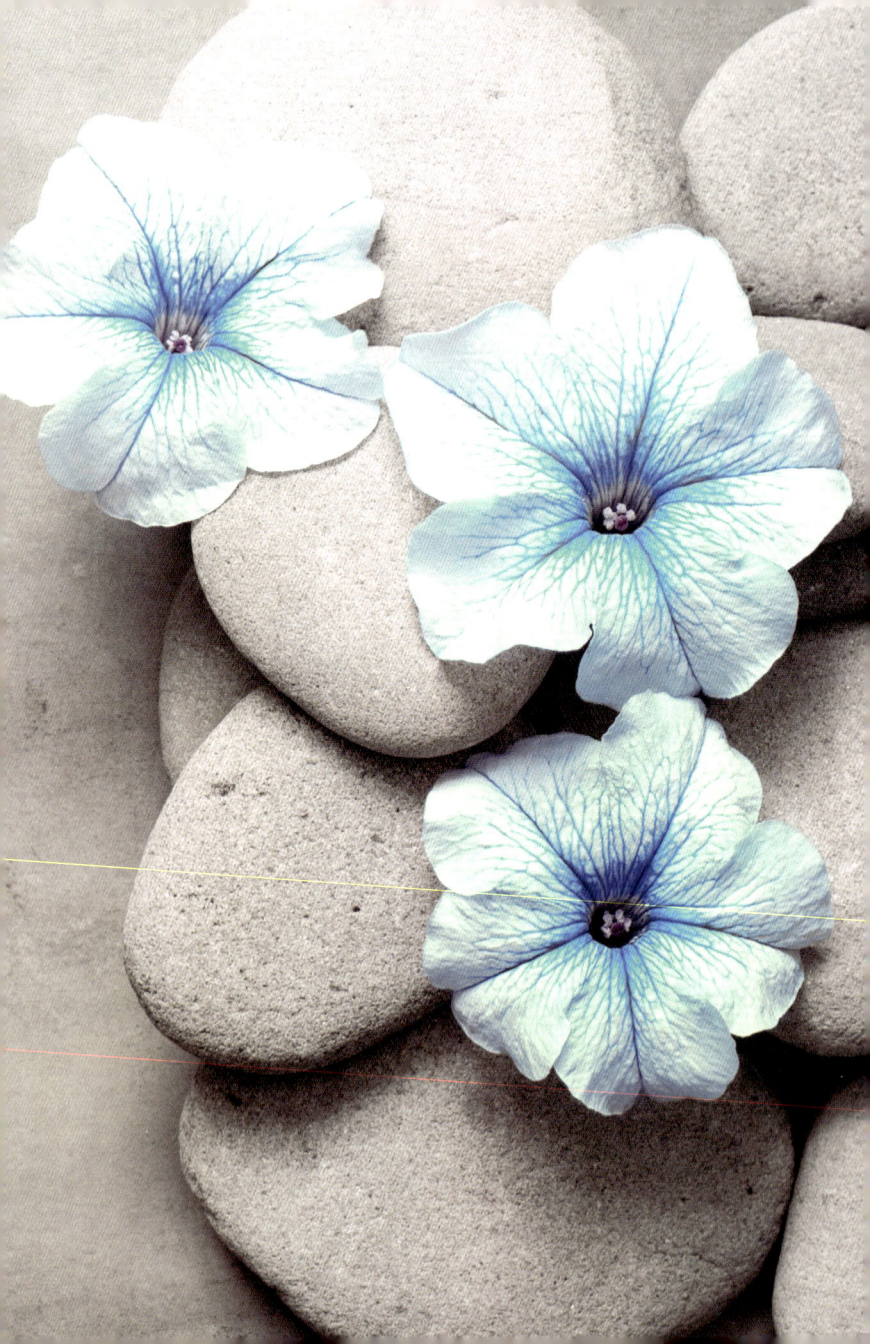

Chapter Two

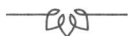

BREATHING
TECHNIQUES
(PRANAYAMA)

The most important part of your meditation practice is something that you do every minute of the day. This chapter will teach you how to use your breath and provide you with advanced breathing techniques to deepen your practice. Learning to focus on and control your breath is a key element of meditation. When done effectively, pranayama breathing will help amplify feelings of peace and calm, move you into a deeper meditative state, and strengthen your connection to your inner self.

Pranayama is a Sanskrit word that roughly translates to *extension of life force*. The word *prana* means *life force* or *breath*, while *ayama* means *to extend or draw out*. In the yoga tradition, breath is believed to carry our life force—our "vital air"—throughout all the parts of our bodies, affecting change in both our physical bodies and energy levels. Maintaining a regular practice of controlling the breath is essential for recharging the body and mind.

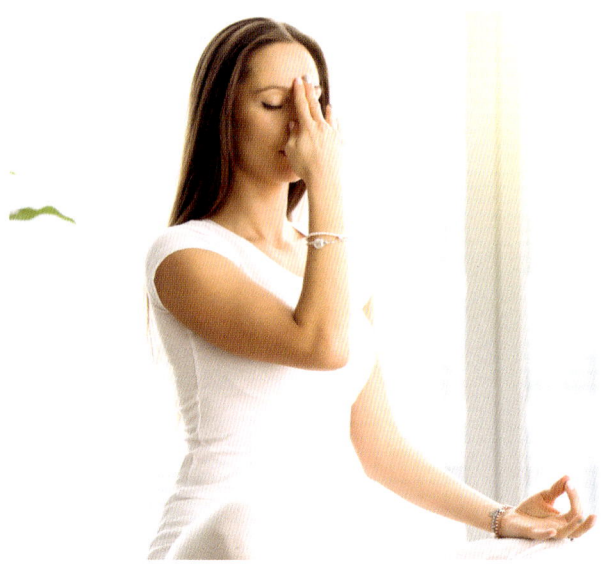

Yoga practitioners believe that the quantity and quality of our life force—our breath—determines our state of mind. When we are not present to our breath—perhaps we are holding it in, taking shallow breaths, or breathing unevenly—it can lead to worry, tension, and stress. When our breath is full, continuous, smooth, and consistent, our mind is calm, enthusiastic, and positive. By practicing simple breathing techniques, it's possible to create a meditation practice you'll want to return to again and again, and to improve your overall experience of life.

Following are five pranayama techniques—listed in order of difficulty—to employ along with the *Calm and Clear* dough to calm the chaos of the mind. Practice your breathing techniques with your eyes closed or focused gently on an object in front of you.

Yoga practitioners believe that the quantity and quality of our life force determines our state of mind.

1. Easy Breath

....

This breathing technique is the simplest to perform. It requires only that you focus your attention on your natural inhales and exhales. There's no need to manipulate your breathing pattern—no counting and no pressure to make your breaths deep, long, or even. Your job at this moment is to pay attention to what's happening in the here and now.

Think of your breath as a messenger reporting on your current physical and energetic condition. If your breathing is short and shallow, you might be worried or tired. Long, deep breaths are indicative of a more peaceful, calm, and relaxed state. Instead of changing your breath, check in to see what it's telling you.

It might be helpful to know that just paying attention to something can often lead to it changing—no big effort required. For instance, you might find that your breath is short and shallow at the beginning of your meditation, but it becomes smoother, longer, and deeper as you focus on it.

How to Practice Easy Breath

1. With your eyes closed or focused on your chosen object, follow your breath as it moves past your nostrils, in through your nose, and down the back of your throat.

2. Allow your chest to rise as your lungs fill with air.

3. Allow the muscles in your abdomen to loosen as your breath fills you up even more.

4. Take a moment at the top of your breath to pause. Then, observe your breath as it exits your body, feeling your belly and your lungs contract, and taking note of the temperature and quality of your breath as it makes its way up through your throat again and out of your mouth.

5. Integrate your *Calm and Clear* dough as you did when learning how to use your mantras. Knead or press your dough into your palms as you inhale, and release on your exhale.

2. Even Breath

....

Another simple breathing technique perfect for calming your mind and body is Even Breath. Practicing this method is as easy as matching the length of each inhale with the following exhale. Your Even Breath should be smooth and quiet, but also intentional and measured. You're going to count silently to yourself to make sure each inhale and exhale match in duration. If you count to four on your inhale, all you have to do is count to four as you exhale.

How to Practice Even Breath

1. Close your eyes or focus gently on your meditation object, and inhale through your nose, counting slowly as your lungs fill full with air.

2. Exhale through your mouth while allowing your jaw to relax and lips to part softly, making sure your exhale is the exact length of your inhale.

3. Empty your lungs.

4. Pause for a moment or two before beginning your next breath cycle.

5. Use your *Calm and Clear* dough by kneading or pressing your dough into your palms as you inhale, and opening your hands on your exhale.

3. One-Two Breath

....

One-Two Breath is a slight twist on Even Breath that's just as easy to perform and highly effective for creating a relaxed mind-body state. When your mind races with worrisome thoughts, distract it with an easy-to-remember pattern to set you on course toward feeling safe and comfortable again. One-Two Breath shifts your focus from something negative toward something neutral. No positive mantra needed here. This method is as easy as multiplying by two.

How to Practice One-Two Breath

(1) With your eyes closed or focused on an object, inhale through your nose while counting silently. Make sure your breath is long and smooth, allowing your lungs and belly to expand. Imagine your entire body filling with air.

(2) Exhale slowly through your mouth, doubling the duration of your inhale. For example, if you count to three during your inhale, make sure your exhale extends for a full six counts.

(3) Pause for a moment at the bottom of each breath cycle. Allowing for emptiness lends itself to creating space in your mind and body. Rest in the stillness of this moment before taking another breath.

(4) With any of your breathing techniques, you can also choose to cradle your *Calm and Clear* dough with both hands at chest level. Instead of kneading your dough, be still and enjoy the scent on each inhale.

You'll learn more about different hand positions in the next chapter.

4. Nadi Shodhana: Alternate Nostril Breathing

....

Now that you've perfected Easy Breath, Even Breath, and One-Two Breath, you're ready for more advanced techniques. Alternate Nostril Breathing or *Nadi Shodhana* is a method that requires a bit more focus and is easily mastered after just a little practice. *Nadi* refers to the channels that run through our body, and *Shodhana* translates to *cleaning* or *purifying*.

The benefits of Nadi Shodhana are numerous. Yoga and meditation practitioners use this technique to calm the nervous system and lower the heart rate, clear energy channels, release toxins, improve concentration, and purify the body.

How to Practice Nadi Shodhana

(1) Sit up nice and tall to create a clear path for energy to flow from the crown of your head down to your seat.

(2) Place your left hand on the thigh or knee or your left leg with your palm upturned. Dough option: Place a *Calm and Clear* dough in your upturned palm and knead it gently in rhythm with your inhales and exhales.

(3) Bring your right hand to your forehead and allow the pointer and middle finger to rest upon your the space between your eyebrows.

(4) Close your eyes or gaze softly upon an object, inhale slowly and deeply through the nose, and exhale through the nose.

(5) Close your right nostril with your right thumb and inhale slowly through the left nostril.

(6) At the end of the inhalation, close the left nostril with your right ring finger and hold your breath for a brief moment.

(7) Release thumb from right nostril and allow the breath to release, emptying the lungs slowly.

(8) At the bottom of your exhale, pause briefly. Inhale through the right side slowly and deeply.

(9) At the top of the inhalation, pause and retain the breath for a moment using thumb and ring finger.

(10) Release ring finger, exhaling through the left nostril. Pause at the bottom of your breath.

(11) Repeat the cycle (steps 5 to 10) for five to ten rounds or for as long as it feels comfortable.

The ratio of your breath should be 1:1, as in Even Breath. As your practice evolves, you will begin to draw deeper breaths, achieving deeper states of relaxation and balance.

5. Ujjayi Breath: Victorious or Ocean Breath

....

Ujjayi Breath is unique because it can relax the body and relieve physical tension while building vitality and internal heat. Ujjayi is commonly translated from Sanskrit as *victorious* and is often referred to as *Ocean Breath* for its sound. When done correctly, this pranayama technique can be both calming and energizing. Ujjayi Breath also energizes the lungs and other vital organs, oxygenates the blood, clarifies thought processes, and detoxes the mind and body.

How to Practice Ujjayi Breath

1. Sit up tall, lengthening the spine to create a clear path for energy. Place hands in prayer position, with palms touching in front of your heart.

2. Dough option: Roll about half of the clarifying rosemary dough into a small ball. Place the ball between the palms and very slowly begin to roll the dough in a circular motion connecting the movement with your breath as you practice.

3. With your eyes closed and your lips sealed, inhale slowly while softly constricting the muscles in the back of the throat. You should notice that this resistance and small effort creates a soothing sound. Too much constriction will create a grasping quality and a rough, grating sound.

4. At the top of your inhale, pause, then release through your nose using the same gentle constriction at the back of the throat. The rhythmic sound should mimic waves rolling in and out.

5. Repeat steps 3 to 4 for two to five minutes or for as long as you feel comfortable.

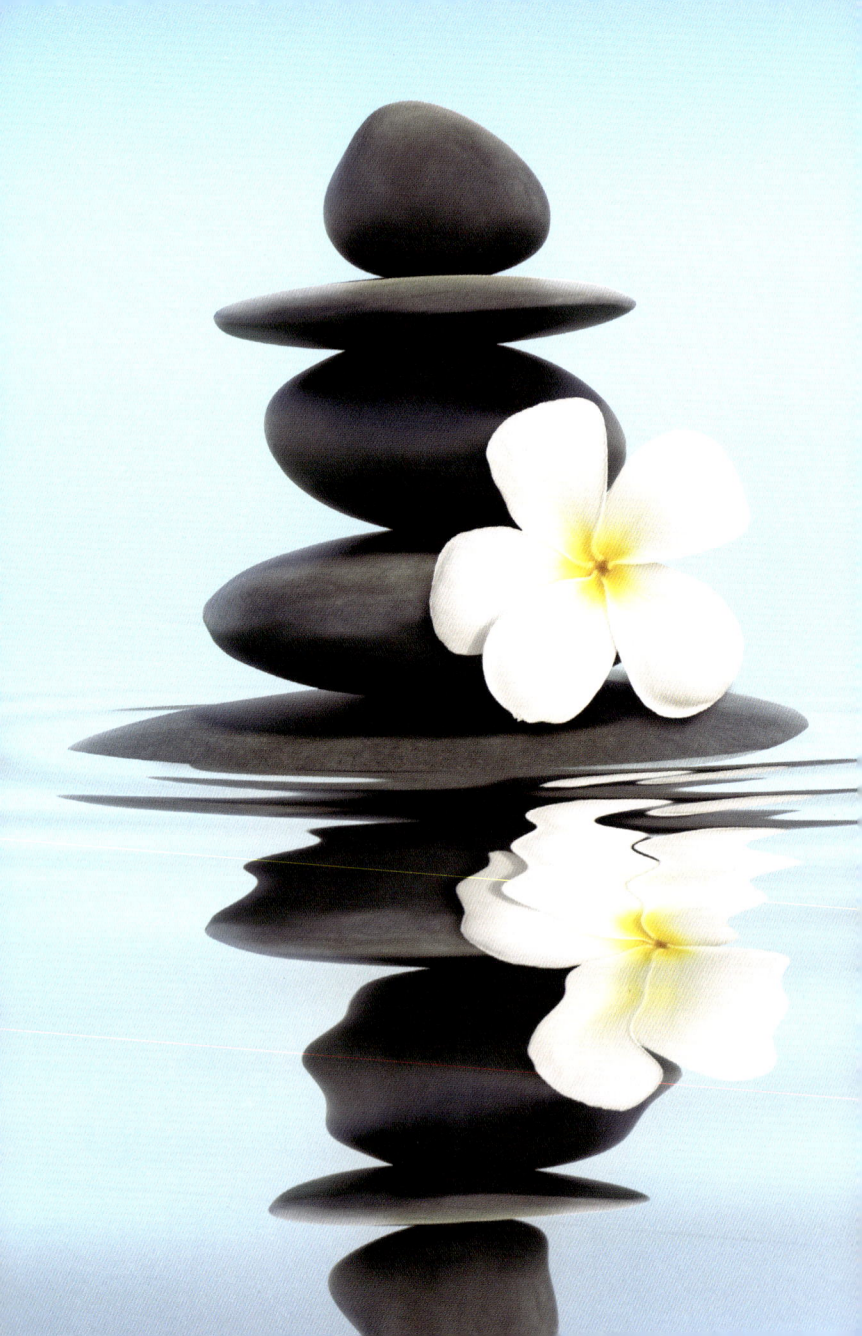

Chapter Three

YOUR MEDITATION PRACTICE

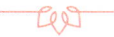

While meditation can undoubtedly take you to the farthest reaches of your psyche and facilitate deep and lasting energetic healing, it's also a straightforward method for connection and relaxation. Meditation allows you to create a pause, to step away from the busyness of your daily schedule and the non-stop activity in your head. It's a way to say to yourself, "I see you, I hear you, and you're worth my time and attention." Meditation allows you to observe the inner workings of your mind while also allowing yourself time to rest and recharge. Televisions must be plugged in to operate. We prioritize recharging our phones. If we don't take the time to plug in and recharge ourselves, we don't work either. Without proper breaks, our brains—and even our spirits—grow tired and lifeless.

C reating a meditation practice that works for you, a time to plug in and recharge, is easy. Despite what many people think, meditation can be practiced successfully by anyone, anywhere, and for any amount of time. All you need is a relatively quiet place to practice and a few moments to focus on your breath. Be encouraged by the fact that you can experience the benefits of meditation immediately. If you pay close attention, you'll notice a shift the very first time you sit down, close your eyes, and focus on your breath. Let that small shift be an indication of the powerful force your future practice will be as you keep practicing.

Unlearn These Three Meditation Myths

. . . .

I t's time to put together all of what you've learned so far and get started on your very own meditation journey. As meditation moves quickly into the mainstream, more people are getting curious about how this mind-body practice can work in their lives. Before we move on, let's dispel three common myths about meditation that may have been keeping you from starting a practice of your own.

Myth 1: Meditation requires that you clear your mind of all thoughts.

Chapter One touched on this myth, but it bears repeating. If the only way to meditate successfully were to clear your mind of all thoughts, it would be a nearly impossible task for anyone to accomplish. Unless you're living a life of solitude on a mountaintop, your whole life dedicated to your meditation practice, turning your mind into a blank slate might be a goal best left by the wayside. A calm and focused mind is the goal, and achieving that goal includes dealing with the thoughts that pop up—not resisting them. Your thoughts are not enemies. Just like your breath, they provide valuable insight into what's going on in the moment, and what needs your attention.

Myth 2: Meditation has to be practiced for a specific amount of time and only at certain times of the day.

Like most people, you're probably busy with your current to-do list. Adding another activity to your schedule—even one meant for self-care—might feel overwhelming. The good news is that while there are many well-established and effective meditation methods that have strict guidelines about when and for how long you should practice, it's also possible to reap significant benefits in just a few short minutes. The benefits of meditation come from the *quality* of your time on your cushion (or chair, or bed) and not the *quantity* of time. We lead busy lives full of responsibilities. Forcing yourself to make time that you don't have is a stress you don't need. Your practice should be something that serves you and meets you where you are right now. Are you able to find a relatively quiet place where you can sit undisturbed for just a few minutes? Can you sit comfortably in a relaxed position long enough to release some tension from your body? Those are the qualities of an effective meditation practice. In time, and at different times, you'll be able to carve out more time for your practice. You'll start to look forward to it, adding it to your daily calendar and maybe even making a special meditation spot in your home (more on that later). If all you have is a few minutes to spare, then that's enough for now.

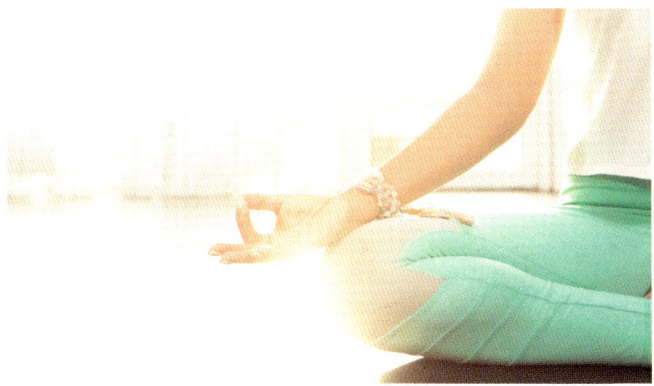

✸ **Myth 3:** You have to be a spiritual or religious person to meditate.

Meditation is a practical tool for managing stress, focusing the mind, and maintaining mind-body harmony. It doesn't belong to any religion or specific philosophy. While many people use meditation as part of their religious practices, there's no requirement to be spiritual or believe in a higher power. Meditation has been used for centuries as a means of maintaining mental, emotional, and physical balance. Countless scientific studies confirm these benefits.[4] No matter what belief system you subscribe—or don't subscribe—to, meditation can help you to achieve balance in your daily life and to achieve even your biggest goals.

If any of these thoughts have kept you from meditating in the past, you should feel more confident about your practice now. There's no reason that you can't integrate meditation into your life in a way that serves you and your wellness goals.

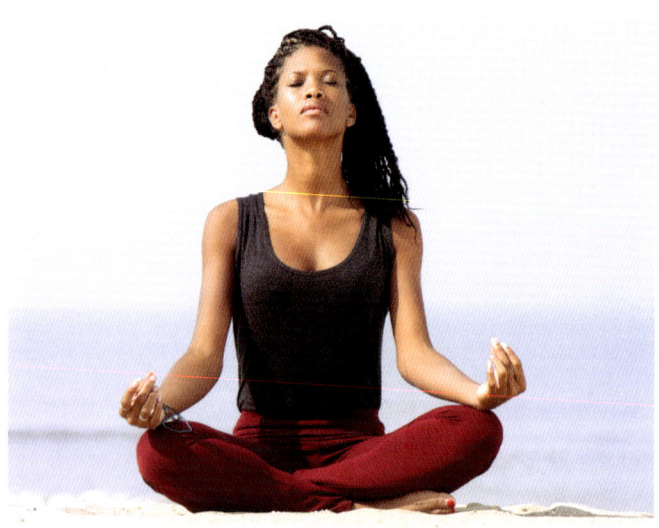

Meditation That Fits Your Life

....

The power of positive mantras and proper breathing techniques will serve as the foundation for your practice. But even as you perfect these methods, keep in mind that all the suggestions in this book are just that—suggestions. Use them as guidelines that you can customize for yourself and your lifestyle. Too much rigidity in any health and wellness journey is unsustainable. Be flexible and forgiving with yourself when learning something new. Keep doing what works for you and leave alone what doesn't. This is your practice to mold into exactly what you want.

Many meditation traditions have precise rules about where, when, and how to meditate. As your practice expands and deepens, feel free to explore more advanced methods. Because traditions like transcendental, Zen, and mindfulness meditation, for instance, involved detailed steps, postures, and other essential elements, it is recommended that you study with a teacher when you begin. Honor tradition, culture, and lineage by learning from those who have mastered the discipline.

For now, let's cover some basic supportive elements of a good practice that will allow you to meditate in a way that best suits your individual needs and situation.

Peace and Quiet

Silence isn't required for a productive meditation experience. A little environmental noise can actually serve you well. We live with constant outside distractions, so learning to navigate just a few during your time in meditation can help you manage stress more easily in the real world. The sounds of nature or the hum of a roadway can be a kind of white noise that makes meditation more accessible. So make it your goal to find a relatively peaceful environment, but don't stress over it being totally silent.

Private Space

Being completely alone isn't necessary, but it is a good idea to find a place where you can sit undisturbed for a little while. Try setting up a dedicated space in your home with a meditation cushion and a scented candle or incense to help set the mood for relaxation and tuning in. Maybe the privacy and comfort of your bedroom would work as the ideal space for you. However, if you share living space with other people and privacy indoors is difficult, consider a spot in nature or the cozy quarters of your car. Meditating in your parked car before work or in between errands can support your energetic wellness on the go. If you like the energy of being around other people, consider participating in group meditation at a local yoga studio or finding a quiet corner of a library to take a few moments for yourself. You can also create personal space in a place occupied by others (for instance, if you work at a cubicle in a crowded office or take public transportation) by closing your eyes and wearing noise-canceling headphones.

Be flexible and forgiving with yourself when learning something new.

A Comfortable Seat

Even sitting for a short amount of time can be uncomfortable, especially if you're dealing with any physical limitations, so it's essential to have the choice of several different meditation poses. It can be challenging to focus on your thoughts when you're feeling pain or discomfort, so decide right now that pain is something you won't tolerate. You're going to learn how to position your body for maximum comfort and so that energy can flow freely, and you can make any one of them your own with minor adjustments. Also, note that stillness during seated meditation is recommended, but that doesn't mean you have to be a statue. A little shimmy now and then to settle into a more comfortable position is perfectly okay.

Meditation Poses to Support Your Practice

....

Sitting in the proper position can make or break your time in meditation. Pain and discomfort should never be tolerated, but getting too comfortable isn't a good idea either. Striking the right balance between being upright and alert and being relaxed and comfortable takes just a little practice.

Your posture doesn't have to be perfect, but there are a few things other than pain that are contraindicated for a successful practice. Avoid slouching or slumping. Meditation is a tool for easing tension and promoting relaxation, but you also want energy and your breath to move throughout your body without obstruction. If you're hunched over in a heap, you're not creating a clear path through which energy can travel. You also don't want to lie completely flat during meditation, unless you intend to fall asleep.

Try out each of the following poses to decide which works best for you. Depending on the purpose of your meditation—to relax, to energize, or to focus—you will find that one position might work better than the others. Let your practice expand and evolve. Don't be afraid to experiment!

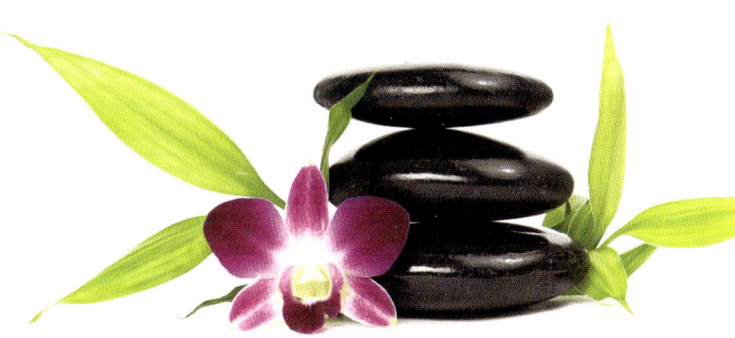

EASY POSE / SUKHASANA

Easy Pose (*Sukhasana* in Sanskrit) is similar to Easy Breath in that it's a natural position that you've probably been doing since childhood. Easy Seat can be practiced almost anywhere. You just need enough space to cross your legs and enough support to maintain good posture. Sitting on a firm, elevated surface like a folded blanket or a meditation cushion can help guide proper alignment of the spine and hips.

How to Get into Easy Pose

1. Sit on the front edge of your blanket with your legs positioned in front of you.

2. Cross your legs so that each foot finds its way under the opposite knee, or so that one shin is in front of the other and the outer edge of each foot is resting comfortably on the floor. Pick whichever position feels more comfortable.

3. Be sure to leave space between your pelvic floor and your legs. There should be no strain in this position. If you feel constricted, make the space larger by moving your shins further away from your body.

4. Sitting up tall, imagine each vertebra of your spine stacked one on top of the other.

5. Lift your shoulders toward your ears on your inhale. Then, on the following exhale, roll your shoulder blades back and down along your spine. This allows your chest to open wide and shine forward. It might also help to imagine a string attached to the crown of your head, pulling you upward. Your chin should be parallel to the floor.

6. Rest your hands on your thighs or knees with palms down for a calming or focus-based meditation, or flipped upward for meditations meant to energize.

Variations on Easy Pose include the Half Lotus and Full Lotus positions. These require one or both of your feet to be brought in to rest sole-upward on the opposite hip crease. The Lotus positions require even greater flexibility and range of motion in the hips, knees, and ankles. Avoid practicing them if you've experienced injury or pain in these areas.

HERO POSE / VIRASANA

Do you want to feel energized, focused, and confident? Hero Pose (*Virasana*) is the perfect, easy alternative to Easy Pose that will allow you to feel strong and rooted during meditation. It can be performed on the floor or seated on a pillow, yoga block, or rolled blanket.

Hero Pose is not recommended if you have knee or hip injuries. Using a prop to elevate your bottom off the floor will help you to feel more at ease in the pose if you have limited flexibility in your knees or hips.

How to Get into Hero Pose

1. Kneel on the floor with your knees together. Separate your calves with a yoga block or rolled blanket if you're attempting Hero Pose for the first time.

2. Part your knees until your thighs are slightly wider than hip-width apart. The tops of your feet should lie flat on the floor.

3. Lower your bottom until you're resting comfortably and safely on your prop or the floor. Allow for about a one-inch gap between the inner edge of each foot and the outer edge of each hip. Make sure you're not experiencing any strain, especially in your knees. Raising your bottom higher with a prop will help ease minor discomfort in your joints.

4. Using the same cues as Easy Pose, with hands clasped above your head, use a full breath cycle to inhale your shoulders up to your ears and exhale your shoulder blades back and down along your spine. You'll find yourself sitting up confidently like a hero.

5. Set your gaze forward, and lift or lower your chin so that it's parallel will the floor.

SEMIRECLINED BOUND ANGLE POSE /
SUPTA BADDHA KONASANA

Sleep isn't usually the goal of meditation, but relaxation often is. And if you happen to be practicing at night before bed or at a time that you'd like to unwind, you certainly don't want to practice an energizing meditation or sit in an energetically charged pose. Semireclined Bound Angle Pose, also known in Sanskrit as *Supta Baddha Konasana*, is a pose well-suited for calming meditations, or for people who have difficulty sitting upright or with their back unsupported. This pose is also ideal for cultivating feelings of openness and vulnerability.

Keeping in mind that you want to feel fully supported while performing this pose, feel free to modify any instruction by adding support props into the mix. For example, placing extra blankets under your knees or behind your head and neck can increase the benefits of the posture for you.

Semireclined Bound Angle Pose is usually performed flat on the floor, but you'll be set up in a semireclined position for meditation. However, if your intention is to drift off into a sweet slumber afterward, lying flat might make that easier.

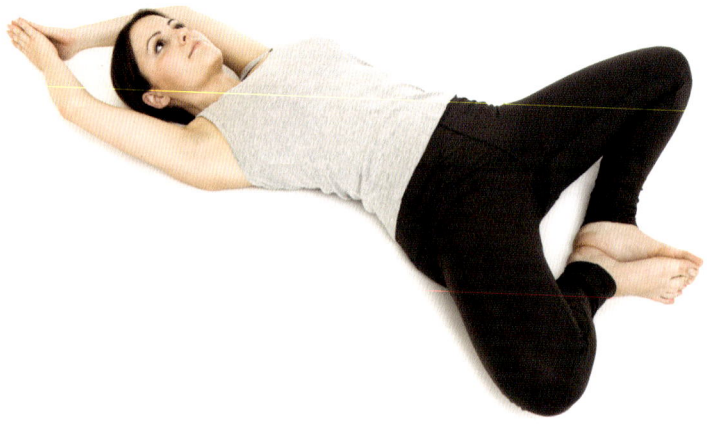

How to Get into Semireclined Bound Angle Pose

(1) Seat yourself on a firm but comfortable surface. Use blankets or a thick mat if you're practicing on a hard floor.

(2) Roll a blanket lengthwise or line up firm pillows to create an elevated surface on which you can rest your spine. Create an angle of 45 degrees or greater between your back and the ground.

(3) With your knees bent and pointed toward the ceiling or sky, place the inner edges of your feet together.

(4) Allow your knees to move away from each other and lower to the floor. Move slowly and stop when you reach the edge of your flexibility. If your knees don't reach the floor (most people's won't unless they're very flexible), place pillows, blankets, or yoga blocks under your legs to prop them up. You should feel a minor stretch in your hips. Allow your muscles to relax and soften on your exhales.

(5) Once your knees are lowered into a comfortable position, make sure the soles of your feet are touching. Adjust your feet closer to or further away from your hips to whatever distance feels most relaxed and natural.

(6) Allow your arms to rest slightly outstretched at your sides with your palms upturned and your fingers outstretched, or above your head in prayer pose.

These are three common seated positions that will serve you well. They aren't the only meditation poses, though. You can meditate at your desk, on the bus, in your car—anywhere you can find a few moments to get quiet, close your eyes, and take a few moments to connect with your breath. Meditating on a chair or other type of seat is also a fantastic option for people with limited mobility or flexibility.

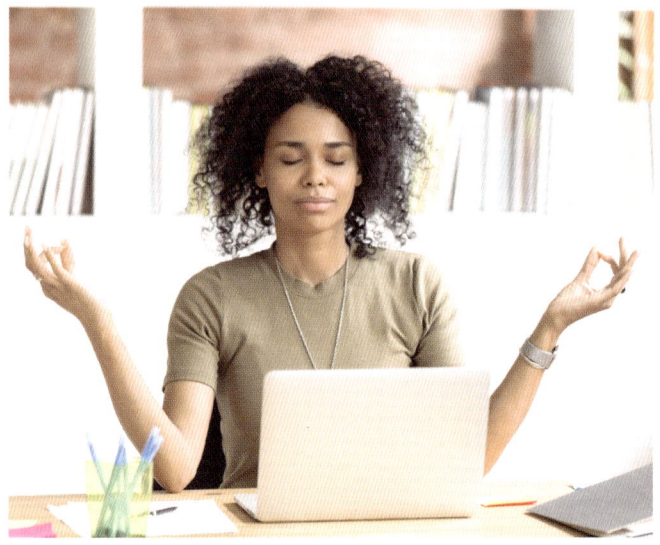

If you prefer practicing in a chair, it's best to make sure your feet are planted firmly on the surface beneath you, and you're sitting up tall, creating a straight path from the crown of your head, down along your spine, and to your seat. Avoid crossing your legs or twisting your body. Place your hands on your knees or near your hip creases, with your palms either turned up or down, or in a mudra.

Picture your breath traveling to all the parts of your body—down your arms to your fingertips, and through your legs to your toes. Make sure the path is free and clear of twists or turns. Doing this will allow you to release tension from every part of your body while allowing positive energy to move through you, restoring peace and vitality wherever it goes.

Mudras: Poses for Your Hands

....

Mudras are symbolic or ritual gestures with origins in Hinduism and Buddhism.[5] A mudra is used to direct energy and may involve individual or all parts of the body. You're probably already familiar with some mudras, even if you were unaware of what you were seeing. Hand mudras are commonly used in meditation and yoga, and representations of the Buddha and Hindu deities are often shown with their hands in mudra positions.

One of the most universally practiced hand gestures is the Anjali or Salutation Mudra, which looks identical to hands in prayer position—palms together and fingers outstretched and connected at the tips. Joining your hands together and holding them in front of your chest (or heart center) is useful for balancing energy between the right and left sides of the body. Place your thumbs on your sternum as a variation to inspire feelings of surrender.

Follow these instructions to perform the Meditation Mudra, Lotus Mudra, and Consciousness Mudra. You'll use your *Calm and Clear* dough to enhance the benefits of each.

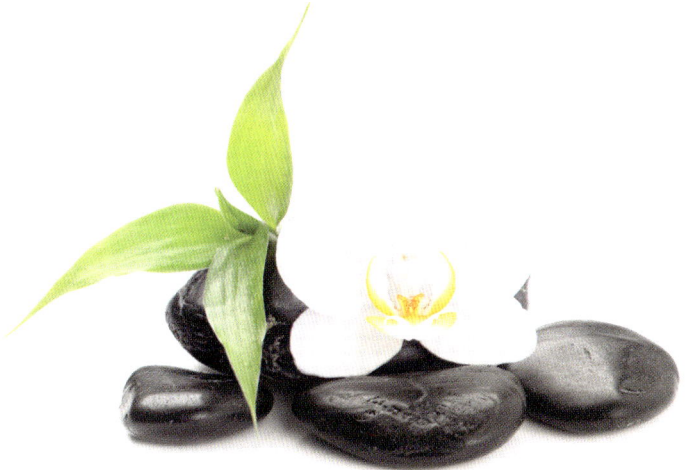

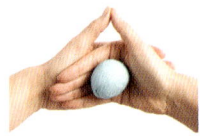

DHYANA MUDRA (MEDITATION OR CHALICE MUDRA)

Perform this two-handed mudra by cradling your left hand with your right (palms facing up and resembling a bowl) and connecting the tips of both thumbs. Rest your hands in your lap. If your legs are crossed, the hand on top should correspond with the leg that's on top. (If your right leg is crossed over your left, place your right hand inside your left hand.) This mudra is for balancing.

>> **HOW TO USE YOUR DOUGH:** *Before settling into meditation and while you're moving through your first breath cycle, roll a medium-size ball of dough (about 2 inches in diameter) between your palms. Open your hands to Dhyana Mudra position, cradling the dough in your open palm. Notice the scent of your dough with every inhale.*

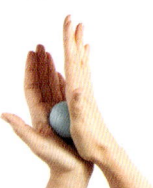

PADMA MUDRA (LOTUS SEAL)

Place your hands in Anjali Mudra in front of your heart center. Slowly, as if you were mimicking a flower opening, spread your fingers apart. Keeping the bottom of your palms and the tips of your pinkies and thumbs connecting, open your hands. Your ring, middle, and index fingers will be outstretched, and your hands will resemble a blooming lotus.

>> **HOW TO USE YOUR DOUGH:** *Place a ball of dough between your palms and press into Anjali Mudra. Open your hands in Padma Mudra, and lift them closer to your face as you inhale. Again, press and close with your exhale (Anjali Mudra), and open and breathe in the scent of the dough on your inhale (Padma Mudra). Continue to open and close your hands during meditation in rhythm with your breath cycles.*

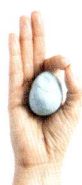

CHIN MUDRA (CONSCIOUSNESS MUDRA)

Connect the tips of your index finger and thumb, forming a small, unbroken circle. Allow the other fingers to remain outstretched. Rest your hands on top of your thighs. Use this mudra for grounding, calming, and focusing.

> **» HOW TO USE YOUR DOUGH:** *Place a small amount of dough in the palm of your hand. On your exhale, bring in your three outstretched fingers to knead the dough. Release and open your fingers into Chin Mudra position on your inhale.*

Your *Calm and Clear* dough can be used with or without your mudras. If you would rather practice with the dough alone, there are myriad options for manipulating and kneading the dough. Here are just a few suggestions:

1. Place the dough on each of your bare thighs, and with your palms turned downward, roll the dough back and forth with each hand, forming two snake-like shapes. Roll the dough toward your hip creases on your inhales and toward your knees on your exhales.

2. Using two hands with fingers outstretched, roll a small ball of dough between your palms. Then, stop and press the dough while curling your fingers over the opposite hand (like a handshake). Roll on your inhales, and press on your exhales.

3. Following your natural breath cycle, press or knead and release your dough to mimic tension and release. Press on your exhales, and release on your inhales.

Now it's time to combine mantra, pranayama, and mudra, and practice your first full-length meditations using your *Calm and Clear* dough. It may be helpful for you to read through the meditations before moving through them. Or, if you have a partner who is willing to help, have them read through the set of steps for each meditation as you practice along. Either of these options will help you get a better idea of the order and pace of the instruction.

Meditation for Peace and Calm

....

Position: Sit in Easy Pose, Semireclined Bound Angle Pose, or comfortably in a chair. This meditation is meant to relax, ground, and center, so being perfectly upright isn't required. Whatever position you choose, make sure there is a straight path from the crown of your head, down your spine, and to the base of your seat or bottom.

Pranayama: Use Even Breath or One-Two Breath for this meditation. These are two of the most straightforward breathing techniques to perform and perfect choices for beginner meditators.

Mantra: "I am safe. I am calm. I am at peace."

Mudra: Choose to keep your hands resting with palms downturned on your knees or thighs or held in the Meditation Mudra. Practice this meditation with your *Calm and Clear* lavender-scented dough.

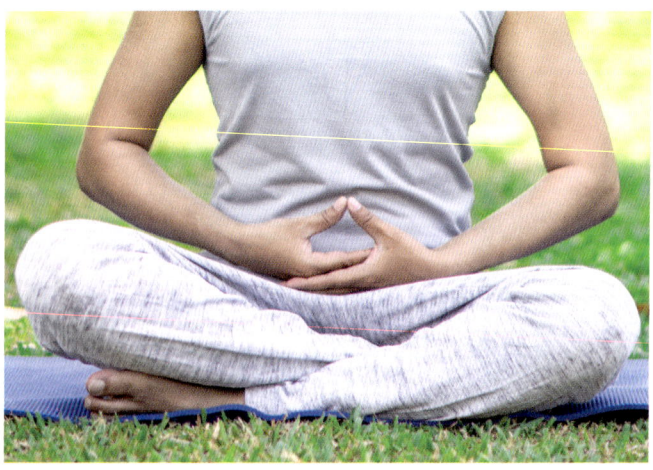

Your Meditation

1. Sitting comfortably with your hands in your chosen mudra or resting position and holding your lavender-scented dough, close your eyes, and focus your attention on your breath.

2. Follow your natural inhales and exhales as your draw air in through your nose and release it from your mouth.

3. Move through a few cycles, observing your breath as it travels past your nostrils, down the back of your throat, into your lungs, and then your belly, and imagine it settling in your seat.

4. Pause for a moment before releasing your breath and following its path up through your body and out of your mouth.

5. Continue breathing using Even Breath or One-Two Breath, counting silently to measure the duration of each inhale and exhale.

6. Once your breathing is smooth and even, recall your mantra to recite silently or out loud with a whisper on your exhale. "I am safe. I am calm. I am at peace."

7. Repeat your mantra for ten full breath cycles while kneading and releasing your dough. Notice the scent drifting through the air and calming you more with each inhale.

8. With each exhale, feel yourself going deeper into a peaceful, Zenlike state. Feel any muscle tension melting away.

9. Continue breathing with Even Breath or One-Two Breath, or return to Easy Breath. Stay here with your eyes closed for as long as feels good.

10. When you're ready, take one last deep inhale and letting-go exhale before opening your eyes and returning to your day.

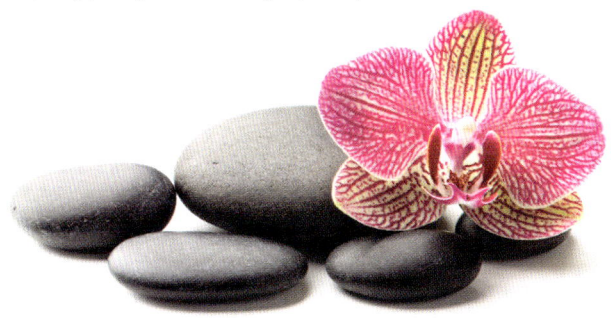

Meditation for Focus and Clarity

....

Position: Easy Pose, Hero Pose, or sitting upright in a chair is recommended for this meditation for mental focus and clarity. Imagine yourself appearing alert and confident with your shoulders broad and open and your chest and face shining forward. Remember the cue to pretend that there's a string attached to the crown of your head, pulling you upward.

Pranayama: Get your circulation moving with Ocean Breath. The sound of your breath will draw your attention inward and keep you focused for the duration of your time in your seat. Your rosemary-scented *Calm and Clear* dough is ideally suited for this energizing meditation.

Mantra: "My mind is clear, and my heart is happy."

Mudra: Choose between two hand positions. You can practice with your hands resting on your knees or thighs with palms upturned to indicate surrender and receiving. Or, for maximum effect, place your hands in Lotus Mudra. As your symbolic lotus opens and blooms, your heart will also open and shine forward, allowing you to receive positive energy through your heart space.

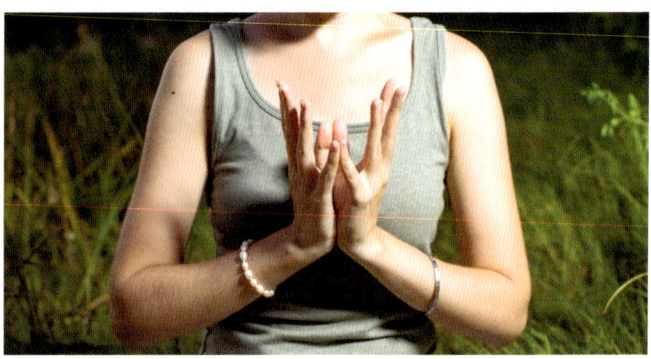

Your Meditation

1. Sitting up nice and tall with your shoulders broad and your chest shining forward, place your hands in your lap or in Lotus Mudra.

2. Breathe into your chest, noticing how it rises on your inhale and falls slowly on your exhale. Continue to follow your breath until it's long, smooth, and even.

3. Now, begin Ocean Breath: Constrict the opening to your throat just a bit so that a little effort is needed to pull in air. Pull air in and push it out, in and out, in and out, making each inhale and exhale match in duration. This should make a sound similar to ocean waves.

4. As you exhale, close your hands to press into and knead your dough, or move from an open Lotus Mudra to a closed Salutation Mudra, pressing the dough between your palms. Inhale and release.

5. You are now breathing with a strong and audible Ocean Breath. The sound of your breathing relaxes and energizes you at the same time. You're sitting up even taller, with your chest shining forward. You feel your heart opening and acting as a portal for receiving waves of positive energy.

6. Every inhale opens your hands like a blooming lotus, and you breathe in the refreshing scent of rosemary. Each exhale allows you to draw in a little, closing your hands to Salutation Mudra and letting your chest fall.

7. Repeat your mantra at the bottom of each of the following seven breath cycles: "My mind is clear, and my heart is happy."

8. Observe how you sit up tall as you pull air into your heart space, feeling vibrant and alive. Notice how relaxed you feel on your exhale, resting just a bit in your seat.

9. After you're finished with your round of seven mantras, return to Easy Breath, and allow your hands to rest in your lap. Remain here for as long as it feels comfortable.

10. When you're ready, open your eyes, smile, and enjoy the rest of your day.

Meditation for Sleep or Deep Relaxation

....

Position: Semireclined Bound Angle Pose is recommended for this meditation. Practice this pose on a yoga mat or blankets the floor, or in bed, propped up by pillows. Consider practicing this variation on this pose that lends itself to a feeling of grounding and safety: Place blankets, hot water bottles, or another weighted object on your lower abdomen, across your hips, or on your knees (only if it feels comfortable; be careful not to overstretch). Many people—especially those who are prone to anxiety or worry—can benefit from this practice. A weighted blanket is also an excellent tool for relaxation meditations and sleep.

Pranayama: A very slow and measured One-Two Breath will help you to fall into a state of deep relaxation. Much like counting sheep, counting the duration of your breaths with full focus will quiet the mind while relieving you of any physical tension.

Mantra: "All is well."

Mudra: Your hands should be free and open for this meditation. Place your lavender-scented dough on a stable surface or the floor next to you. Maybe you'll want to spend a few moments kneading your dough and taking in the soothing scent before beginning your practice. Allow your arms to fall by your sides with palms upturned and fingers outstretched but relaxed. Alternatively, you can place one hand (palm down) right below your navel and your other hand on your heart space.

Your Meditation

① Settling into your deeply comfortable Semireclined Bound Angle Pose, close your eyes, and bring your attention to your smooth, long, deep inhales and exhales.

② Allow your chest and belly to rise and fall as your body fills with life force and returns peaceful energy to the space around you.

③ Observe how each part of your body feels. Scan your body from crown to toes, noticing any tension in your muscles.

④ Release the muscles in your forehead and behind your eyes. Allow your jaw to soften and your lips to part. Relax your shoulders and your arms. Let your body sink into the surface beneath you. Relax your hips, and let your legs be heavy.

⑤ Imagine your energy being drawn down past the materials supporting you, through the floor, into the ground, and toward the center of the earth. You feel grounded, rooted, safe, and secure.

⑥ Start counting the duration of your inhales and exhales. Take the time to breathe in slowly, counting how many seconds it takes to fill your lungs. Then, double the number of seconds for your exhale.

⑦ At the bottom of your exhale, pause for a moment to repeat your mantra either silently or out loud with a whisper. "All is well."

⑧ Continue to count and breathe. Notice how your breath becomes longer, deeper, and smoother with hardly any effort at all. Notice how calm and relaxed you feel in your body as you repeat, "All is well."

⑨ There is no time limit for this meditation. Stay here for as long as you'd like or until you fall fast asleep. Know that treating yourself to this practice before bed sets you up for a restful night's sleep, pleasant dreams, and an even better tomorrow.

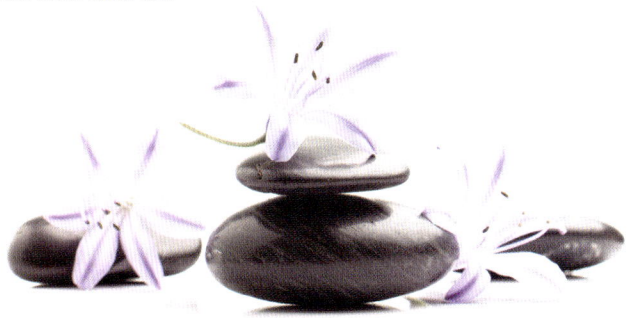

Make Meditation Your Own

....

What you read on these pages is merely the beginning of your journey and only a drop in the mindfulness ocean. It's simply a humble offering of what might work for you. There are no rules set in stone or an assertion that there is one perfect way to approach meditation. There are as many ways to meditate as there are people on this planet. You can't do it wrong, and there are infinite ways to do it right.

Take what you've learned and create a practice of peace, clarity, and joy that is indeed yours. Mix and match the mantras, mudras, and breathing techniques to build meditations that work just for you and your lifestyle. Add new methods to your toolkit through further research. There's a wealth of knowledge out there that will keep you learning and growing for a lifetime. Just know that what you started here can fully support you in deep relaxation, improved mental clarity, and perfect focus.

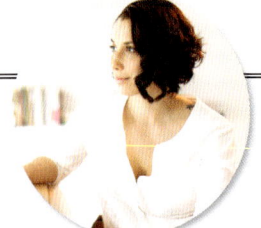

About the Author

Rebekah "Bex" Borucki, founder of BexLife® and the Blissed In® wellness movement, is a mother of five, TV host, meditation guide, best-selling author, birth doula, and life transformation and resilience coach. Visit BexLife.com to connect with Rebekah and her online community.

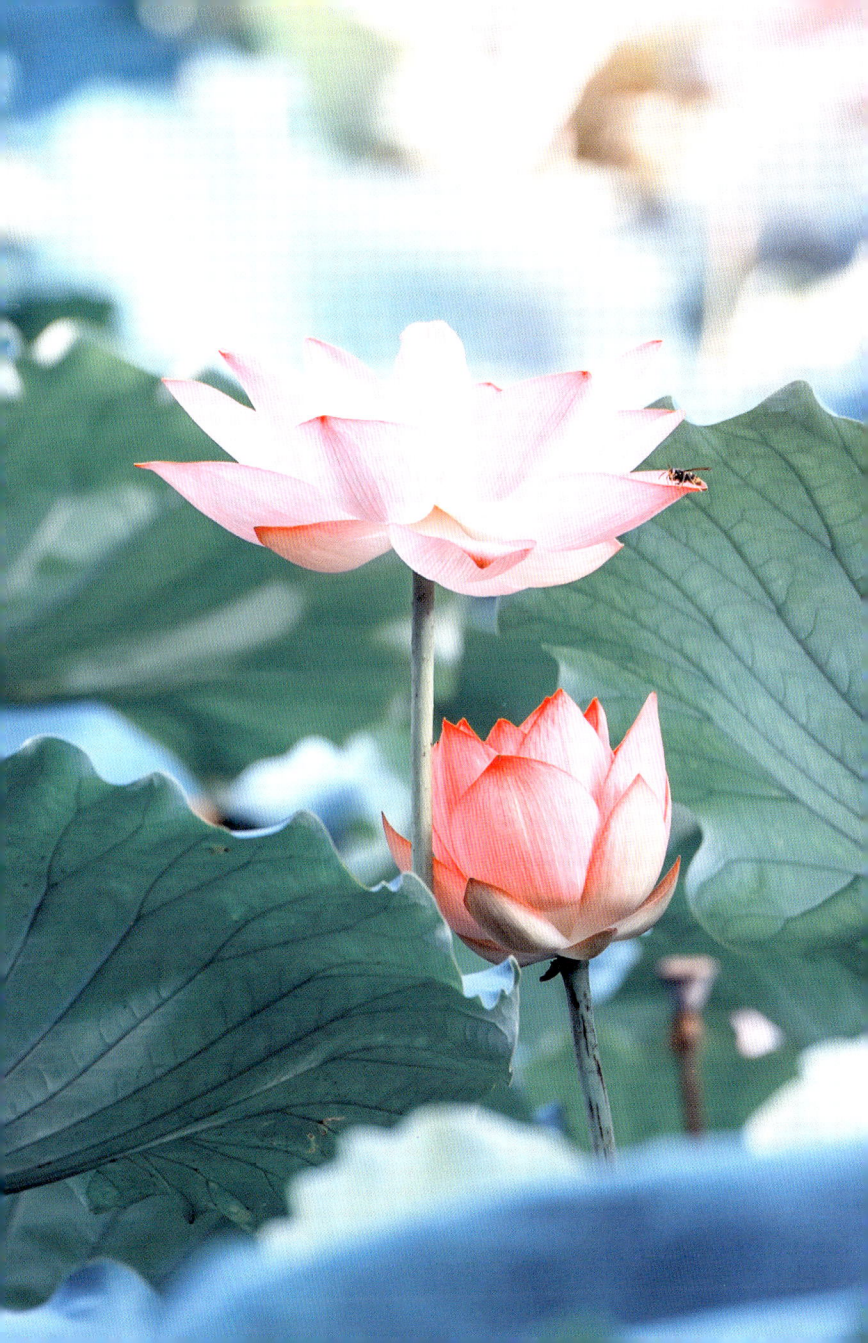

Notes

. . . .

1 "What's in a Mantra?" Gaia.com. January 29, 2013. http://gaia.com/article/whats-mantra

2 Field, Tiffany, PhD, Miguel Diego, Maria Hernandez-Reif, Wendy Cisneros, Larissa Feijo, Yanexy Vera, Karla Gil, Diana Grina, and Qing Claire He. "Lavender Fragrance Cleansing Gel Effects on Relaxation." *International Journal of Neuroscience*, Volume 115, 2005 - Issue 2 (April 2004): 207-222. https://doi.org/10.1080/00207450590519175

3 Van Tulleken, Chris. "What does rosemary do to your brain?" *BBC News Magazine*. July 15, 2015. https://www.bbc.com/news/magazine-33519453

4 Goyal, Madhav. Sonal Singh, Erica M. S. Sibinga, Neda F. Gould, Anastasia Rowland-Seymour, Ritu Sharma, Zackary Berger, et al. "Meditation Programs for Psychological Stress and Well-being." *JAMA Intern Med*. 2014;174(3):357-368. doi:10.1001/jamainternmed.2013.13018

5 McCord, Andy. "The Secret Language of Hands in Indian Iconography." Smithsonian Journeys Quarterly (itals). February 17, 2016. https://www.smithsonianmag.com/travel/india-hand-gestures-mudra-180958089/